Text Copyright © 2017 by Michelle Bailey

All rights reserved. No part of this guide may be reproduced in any form without permission in writing from the publisher except in the case of brief quotations embodied in critical articles or reviews.

Legal & Disclaimer

The information contained in this book is not designed to replace or take the place of any form of medicine or professional medical advice. The information in this book has been provided for educational and entertainment purposes only.

The information contained in this book has been compiled from sources deemed reliable, and it is accurate to the best of the Author's knowledge; however, the Author cannot guarantee its accuracy and validity and cannot be held liable for any errors or omissions. Changes are periodically made to this book. You must consult your doctor or get professional medical advice before using any of the suggested remedies, techniques, or information in this book.

Upon using the information contained in this book, you agree to hold harmless the Author from and against any damages, costs, and expenses, including any legal fees potentially resulting from the application of any of the information provided by this guide. This disclaimer applies to any damages or injury caused by the use and application, whether directly or indirectly, of any advice or information presented, whether for breach of contract, tort, negligence, personal injury, criminal intent, or under any other cause of action.

You agree to accept all risks of using the information presented inside this book. You need to consult a professional medical practitioner in order to ensure you are both able and healthy enough to participate in this program.

Table of Contents

INTRODUCTION 5

CHAPTER 1 WHAT EXACTLY IS DIABETES? 8
- Metabolism and Blood Sugar 9
- The Different Types of Diabetes 11
- What can Diabetes do to You? 15
- Myths & Facts 22

CHAPTER 2 ARE YOU AT RISK? 29
- Why Prevention Matters 36
- Can You Really Diabetes-Proof Your Life? 38
- When to see a Doctor 40

CHAPTER 3 WEIGHT MANAGEMENT MADE EASY 45
- Calculating Your BMI 46
- Your Waistline, Your Lifeline 48
- The No Fuss Diet 49

CHAPTER 4 ALL YOU NEED TO KNOW ABOUT THE GLYCEMIC INDEX 57
- Low vs. High GI 59
- The Carbohydrates Debate 63
- The Glycemic Load on your Blood Sugar 67
- Calculating the Glycemic Load 68

CHAPTER 5 MAKING SENSE OF CARBOHYDRATES 70
- Portion Control Made Easy 72
- Get Moving! 78
- Coach, Not Coax, Yourself into Fitness 80
- No More Excuses! 81

WHAT IS BEST FOR ME? 83
YOUR DIABETES CONTROL AND PREVENTION CHEAT SHEET 87
BEST FOODS TO GO WITH CARBOHYDRATES 90
CONCLUSION **97**

INTRODUCTION

If you are able to lead a considerably normal life, eat anything you desire, have no mobility limitations, are of a healthy body weight and are not on any long-term medication - you can be considered a perfectly healthy individual. If that's the case, diabetes is probably the least of your worries. At least not until you enter your fifties and the body's wear-and-tear begin to show its cumulative effect. But you could not be further from the truth.

Diabetes Mellitus - the groups of metabolic disorders affecting the body's use of glucose - is one of the most common conditions affecting a significant chunk of the world's population. It does not help that the typical modern lifestyle continues to perpetuate habits which increases one's diabetes risk factors, from a diet filled with processed foods to long desk-bound working hours. For all you know, you could be unknowingly setting the stage for the disease to eventually take over your life, because of the seemingly harmless lifestyle choices you make each day.

As you are about to learn in this volume, regardless of your how high or low your diabetes risk factor is, it is never too late and certainly doesn't hurt to diabetes-proof your life. That's because while diabetes is a treatable and manageable condition, it is also preventable in most cases. Plus, living with diabetes is no walk in the park; a host of serious and even deadly complications can develop when a diagnosis is made and the condition is poorly managed.

The information in this book is mainly geared toward individuals with potentially high risk for developing diabetes, and wish to make sensible changes to their lives to lower their risk. It is not intended as a substitute to proper medical care and advice from a qualified healthcare professional. So, by all means, please consult a physician if you or someone you know could be suffering from symptoms of diabetes. What you have here is a layperson's guide to understanding diabetes as a condition, how it can affect one's quality of life and most importantly, what you can do in your day-to-day life to lower your risk and prevent it. With knowledge, you will be better able to gauge your diabetes risk factors, and perhaps have a more informed discussion with your doctor.

If you have been diagnosed and living with diabetes, there is also plenty of information in these pages that would be beneficial to you, especially the information in chapters 3 to 5. Because with a disease like diabetes that is very much part of your life, the more you know, the more empowered you will be and the less helpless you will feel against it.

Because diabetes affects the body chemistry, you will learn about simple dietary and lifestyle changes that can go a long way in not only preventing diabetes, but also help you maintain optimal weight and significantly improve your overall well-being. Regardless of your current state of health, it pays to not take it for granted.

CHAPTER 1

WHAT EXACTLY IS DIABETES?

Despite its prevalence today, diabetes is far from a new disease. In fact, the earliest known account was first documented in the second century AD by the Greek physician, Aretus the Cappadocian. The physician described a condition called <u>diabainein</u>, where patients were observed to be frequently urinating (a symptom of diabetes; more on this later). The disease had also been documented in ancient China, where it was noted that ants would be attracted to the urine of a person who has the "Sweet Urine Disease".

So, what exactly is this condition called Diabetes Mellitus? How can one end up developing it? Is it treatable? More importantly, how can you prevent it? Before you can adopt the essential lifestyle habits to minimize your own risk, you have to first thoroughly understand of what the disease is, and what goes on in the body' system when a person becomes diabetic.

Metabolism and Blood Sugar

In a nutshell, diabetes is a group of metabolic diseases characterized by high levels of glucose. Metabolism is the chemical reaction that occurs when the body breaks down the food we consume to be used for energy and growth. When foods are digested, they are broken down into the main source of body fuel known as glucose, a form of sugar in the blood (hence, it is also known as blood sugar). The glucose then makes its way into the bloodstream to be used by the body's cells. However, the cells cannot absorb glucose without the presence of a hormone known as insulin, which is produced by the pancreas.

After eating, an adequate amount of insulin is released by pancreas to move the glucose in the blood into the cells. In healthy individuals, insulin regulates glucose levels by ensuring the rate of glucose produced by the liver matches the rate use by the body's cells. Once the glucose are absorbed by the cells, blood sugar levels would drop.

In the case of a diabetic, the pancreas does not produce enough insulin or the body cells do not respond properly to the hormone - or in certain cases, both - resulting in hyperglycemia, a condition where a person's blood sugar is higher than normal. The excess glucose would then be release out of the body in the urine. So, although the blood has plenty of glucose, the cells are not getting the needed fuel for energy and growth. If left untreated or uncontrolled, this will eventually lead to a host of health complications.

Now that you know what goes on in the body that leads to diabetes, we shall look at the different types of metabolic diseases that fall into this group, their causes and what one can do to manage or prevent them.

The Different Types of Diabetes

No diabetes case is the same, and thus should one be diagnosed with diabetes, effective management of the condition is an individualistic approach under the guidance of a health care professional. As such, it is difficult to pinpoint a single cause for diabetes, because it is often a combination of several factors and it varies for each individual. There are three different types of diabetes, each vary considerably in terms of cause. Let's look at each one of them:

Type 1 Diabetes

Also referred to as juvenile diabetes, insulin-dependent diabetes or early onset diabetes, Type 1 diabetes is essentially an autoimmune reaction. Like all autoimmune disorders, it is caused by the immune system attacking and destroying the body's cells which it is supposed to protect. In Type 1 diabetes, cells of the pancreas responsible for producing insulin is being destroyed by the immune system, leaving the body without sufficient insulin to function normally.

The cause of Type 1 diabetes is often attributed to genetics. Additionally, viral or bacterial infection, chemical toxins found in food and other unidentified components that could trigger autoimmune reactions are also suspected as likely causes. This type of diabetes usually develops in early adulthood, before the age of 40. It is also possible for one to be diagnosed with Type 1 as young as in their teens.

This is the rarer type of diabetes, accounting for approximately only 10% of all diabetes cases worldwide. Unfortunately, Type 1 diabetes is also a lifelong condition that currently has no known preventable measure or cure. Patients will need to be given insulin injections for the rest of their life, monitor their blood sugar with regular blood tests and follow a specific diet to maintain their well-being (more on this in Chapter 3).

Type 2 Diabetes

The most common type of diabetes, making up approximately 90% of all cases, happens when the body does not produce enough insulin or the cells of the body is insulin resistant. Multiple factors can cause Type 2 diabetes, most notably a family history with the disease. But your genetics is not destiny though, because Type 2 diabetes is generally regarded as resulting from prolonged poor lifestyle choices. Overweight individuals who lead a sedentary lifestyle with unhealthy eating habits are at the highest risk of developing this form of diabetes, especially as they get older.

With early diagnosis and action, it is possible for individuals to control their Type 2 diabetes symptoms with dietary changes, regular exercise, losing weight and monitoring their blood sugar levels. However, the disease is usually progressive, and over time, one would have to be on medication to make up for the insulin deficiency.

On the plus side, Type 2 diabetes is very much preventable by maintaining an active lifestyle, and sensible eating habits.

Prediabetes

If one's blood sugar levels are higher than normal, but not high enough to be considered as diabetic, the condition is known as prediabetes. Although not a full-fledged disease, it can cause heart and blood circulation complications. It is an indicator that body cells are becoming insulin resistant. Prediabetes is also considered a precursor to Type 2 diabetes and has a high likelihood of progressing into the disease left unchecked.

Fortunately, prediabetes does not have to turn into Type 2 and it can be reversed with the right nutrition and guidance from a doctor. It does, however, take diligent effort on the individual's part. If you have been diagnosed with prediabetes, it should be a wakeup call to get yourself on a diabetes prevention immediately, if you want to stop the disease in its tracks.

Gestational Diabetes

Little is known about what can cause a type of diabetes that can occur during pregnancy, known as Gestational diabetes, the condition where an expecting mother has very high levels of glucose because their bodies are unable to produce enough insulin. Studies by the National Institute of Health and Harvard University found that women with a pre-pregnancy diet that is high in cholesterol and animal fat are at much higher risk.

Diagnosis for this kind of diabetes has to be made during pregnancy. If left undiagnosed and uncontrolled, there is a risk of birthing complications and the baby may be born with a heavy birth weight. Exercise and diet can help with managing gestational diabetes, although come patients will need medication.

What can Diabetes do to You?

There is a common misconception that living with diabetes is just a nuisance, but it is not as serious compared to other long-term conditions like cardiovascular diseases. Sure, having to watch what you eat, monitor your blood sugar and probably be dependent on insulin shots can be an inconvenience. But if left unchecked, diabetes is far from a safe condition. For starters, being diabetic is estimated to shorten one's life expectancy by an average of five to ten years. There is also host of serious health issues that can result from it. Let's look a list of possible complications linked to poorly managed diabetes in detail:

Kidney Disease

When the body is unable to eliminate the waste products of sugar and starches, it causes the blood sugar to rise and also makes it difficult for protein to pass through. If diabetes remained uncontrolled, the kidneys have to work harder than usual, filtering too much blood and begin leaking. This then leads to a build-up of waste material in the blood. Eventually, like any overworked organ, the kidneys give out and the person would have to be put on dialysis, whereby a machine would have to perform the functions of the kidneys. In the worst case scenario, a kidney transplant may be needed, since we cannot live without the vital bean-shaped organs.

Cardiovascular Diseases

Diabetics have twice the likelihood of suffering from a heart attack or stroke than non-diabetics. This is due to blood vessels being damaged by high amounts of glucose in the blood, resulting in the blood vessels working harder to pump blood from the heart throughout the body. When it comes to heart health, keeping your cholesterol and blood pressure in check is important for everyone, but it is imperative for diabetics because the presence of excess glucose can weakened the blood vessels. High blood pressure (hypertension) in particular is common among diabetics, and this in itself increases the risk of heart attack, stroke, kidney troubles and eye problems.

In fact, diabetes itself is a risk factor for cardiovascular diseases. They often go hand in hand and have a lot of general risk factors in common, such as obesity and high levels of bad cholesterol. Hence, to prevent diabetes is to prevent heart diseases down the line.

Retinopathy (Eye Complications)
When the tiny blood vessels in the retina has too much

glucose, they gradually weaken and become damaged, leading to problems like blurry vision, pain or pressure in the eyes, dark spots in front of the eyes, and peripheral vision troubles. Besides retinopathy, diabetics are also at risk of other eye complications like cataracts and glaucoma. Cataracts are easily curable with surgery, but glaucoma can lead to blindness if not treated fast. Eye complications among diabetic take a long time to develop. So, it is never too late begin early care and prevention with the help of an ophthalmologist, if a person is diagnosed with diabetes.

Sexual Dysfunction

Because the body responds to sexual stimuli through the nerves, sexual response lessens as high amounts of glucose progressively damages the nerves. Sexual dysfunction affect both men and women, albeit differently. For men, erectile dysfunction is both a symptom and result of diabetes. But that's not where it stops! A diabetic man can also experience retrograde ejaculation, which more potentially dangerous condition where semen enters the bladder instead of being dispelled out of the penis during ejaculation. Meanwhile, women often experience dryness that can make intercourse painful, due to lack of response in the nerve cells within the vagina. As the disease progresses, many diabetics, both male and female, express less interest in sex.

Many people are hesitant to seek help when it comes to problems relating to their sexual relations out of embarrassment. But the dip in sex drive could lead to one's self-esteem taking a nosedive, making it likely for a person to fall into depression. Other than possibly putting a dent in one's marriage, sexual dysfunction may seem like the least harmful of all diabetes-related complications. Even so, it is worth noting whether the change in your sex drive has a medical implication.

Infections and Foot Complications
High blood sugar levels adversely affects the central nervous system and also the nerves in various parts of the body over time. The legs and feet are most affected here, since it is furthest from the brain. One of these complications is

Peripheral Arterial Disease (PAD), which causes pain and tingling sensations in the legs, and sometimes makes walking difficult.

Nerve damage can cause a loss of sensation and feelings in the feet. Hence, a person with poorly controlled diabetes can injure their feet without feeling it and getting it treated immediately, resulting in a slow healing wound or blister.

Since high glucose also makes one more prone to all sorts of infections. This is especially worrisome if an open wound on the foot becomes infected as it can lead to gangrene. If a diabetic sustained injury to the foot, it is critical to seek immediate medical attention to prevent the wound from becoming infected. Gangrene is deadly, and once it sets in, the only course of treatment is amputation. Needless to say, foot complications are the most feared outcome for diabetics.

HHNS (Hyperosmolar Hyperglycemic Nonketotic Syndrome)

When blood sugar levels shoot up too high, the body will desperately try to expel the excess sugar by passing it into the urine. You will end up going to the bathroom more frequent than usual, feeling extremely thirsty and have dark colored urine. HHNS can happen to diabetics with either Type 1 or 2, but it is more common among those with Type 2. Elderly individuals with diabetes are more susceptible to this complication, and it is normally triggered by something else like an illness or infection that causes rapid glucose spikes.

HHNS is a medical emergency, and it's the diabetes complication that can cause death. It that may develop over several days or even weeks. Thus, early signs of it - extreme thirst, frequent urination and dark urine - should not be ignored is a person is diabetic. If not attended immediately, HHNS can cause severe dehydration that will lead to seizures, coma, and eventually death.

But it Doesn't Have to be This Way!

These diabetes-linked complications are not meant to scare

you, but rather to inform you of what's at stake if diabetes becomes part of your life. The good news is - even for those who are living with diabetes - all those aforementioned complications are very much avoidable. All of them stemmed from the body not processing glucose normally. With proper self-care through diet and exercise, along with careful monitoring of one's blood sugar and following doctor's orders, it's possible to prevent diabetes from compromising your quality of life - for diabetics and non-diabetics alike. Next, we shall demystify some long-standing misinformation about diabetes.

Myths & Facts

If you are looking for information on how to prevent or manage diabetes, there are no shortages of unsubstantiated beliefs, old wives tales and straight up misinformation being passed around as presumed facts about the disease. Even when your goal is prevention, knowing how to separate facts from false information can be helpful, especially if you have acquaintances and loved-ones who are diabetic or prediabetic. So, before we get to how you can tweak your lifestyle and minimize your diabetes risk, here are a number of myths that need to be addressed:

You are more likely to become diabetic someday, if you keep eating a lot of sugary foods. - You've probably heard of this from your parents, just as soon as you were old enough as a child to have a sketchy understanding of what diabetes is. This has a tiny ounce of truth. A diet high in sugar and calories can lead to weight gain and obesity which - coupled with family history - is a huge risk factor for developing Type 2 diabetes down the line. However, someone can develop Type 1 diabetes from an autoimmune reaction, whether or not they are fond of sweet treats. So, indulging your sweet tooth in moderation won't hurt, as long as you maintain a predominantly healthy and balanced diet.

You will eventually become diabetic if you are overweight. - Much like the "curd your sweet tooth" advice, this is very much a myth. Being overweight doesn't set one on a path to

Type 2 diabetes, any more than maintaining optimal weight guarantees you will be free of the disease. That's because the cause of diabetes cannot be narrowed down to a single factor. There are many overweight individuals who did not develop diabetes.

Diabetic children can eventually outgrow it. - Sadly, unless a cure is found someday soon, the insulin-producing cells in the pancreas have been destroyed for children with Type 1 diabetes and nothing can reverse that. That means they will need to be on insulin for the rest of their lives.

Only older people have to be concerned about developing diabetes. - Our immune system weakens with age, thus making us more susceptible to illnesses. So, while age is another significant diabetes risk factor, like obesity, it is not an inevitability. In fact, in recent decades, experts have noticed a steady rise in Type 2 diabetes among the younger demographic, including children and teenagers. This is believed to be due to the increase in childhood obesity from poor diet and lack of physical activity.

Diabetics need to adhere to a special diet. - The diet recommended by nutritionists and doctors for diabetics is in fact nothing more than a balanced diet. It contains plenty of fruits, vegetables and whole grains, while being low in salt, sugar and unhealthy fats - a diet everyone should be following for their well-being, diabetic or not. It's just that for diabetics, it is more imperative to watch one's diet. You will learn all about healthy dietary practices in Chapter 3.

Chocolates, candies and sweet desserts should be off limits if you are diabetic. - As long as you lead a healthy lifestyle, with plenty of exercise and good eating habits, the moderate sugary indulgence won't kill you, even as a diabetic.

Diabetics are not allowed to eat bread, pasta and potatoes. - In moderate portions, starchy foods are safe. Wholegrain starchy foods are always the better option, even for non-diabetics.

High blood sugar levels do not necessarily mean you are diabetic. - Certain illnesses, steroids, and mental stress can cause temporary rise in blood sugar levels for non-diabetics, but that should pass after a reasonable amount of time. With that said, having high glucose levels are never normal nor okay for anyone! In fact, that should be a cue to get tested for diabetes.

You will know it when your blood sugars are to high or low. - There are definitely symptoms that indicate your blood sugar is too high or low, but that' snot always the case. That's because there has to be significant fluctuating in glucose levels for symptoms to be felt The only way you can be sure if you blood-sugar is optimal is to have them tested regularly.

If I have to go on insulin, it means my diabetes is at its worst. - When diet and other non-insulin diabetes drugs do not provide enough control for one's condition, insulin becomes necessary. Because no case of diabetes is exactly the same, needing to be on insulin usually does not usually mean a person is at the end of the line with the disease. Unlike cancer and other terminal illnesses, diabetes does not have stages of progression.

Diabetes weakens your immune system. - A diabetic is no more susceptible to illness than others. But since certain illnesses and medication can cause blood sugar to fluctuate, when a diabetic gets sick, such as catching a cold, it can make their condition harder to control and thus putting them at higher risk of complications.

Diabetics should not exercise. - This myth most likely stemmed from the baseless theory that because a person with diabetes is deprived of body fuel from glucose, they should not exhaust themselves with vigorous physical activities. Regular exercise and weight management is extremely important for diabetics and maintaining a healthy workout routine is beneficial for keeping the pounds off. Plus, exercising improves cardiovascular health, relieves stress and helps regulate blood sugar. We will cover exercising in Chapter 5.

Diabetes is transmittable. - The only way for diabetes to be passed on is from a parent to their offspring, through their genes. Even so, that would only put one at higher risk of diabetes, and does not seal their fate with the disease. Lastly, diabetes is a disease that has to do with the body chemistry. It is not caused by a contagious virus or bacteria and hence not transmittable in the way a cold would.

Having known what diabetes is and is not, and what can happen from it, perhaps you can see why there is no better time to begin some sort of diabetes prevention plan. In the following chapter, you will learn to gauge your risk factor, and find out how to realistically minimize your chances of developing the disease.

CHAPTER 2

ARE YOU AT RISK?

If the risk for diabetes can be narrowed down to one thing, it would be diet - one that is high in sugar, starch, and simple carbohydrates, while being low in nutrients. Poor eating habits, when coupled with an inactive lifestyle, leads to weight gain. In fact, the diabetes epidemic has been observed to mirror the obesity epidemic in countries like America and the United Kingdom, where the populations' staple diet consists fast and processed food.

Furthermore, being overweight is not only a huge risk factor for diabetes, but for plenty of diseases as well and a number of them actually has links to diabetes, either as a cause or as a result of.

As you use the information here to make an assessment of your own susceptibility to the disease, it should be noted that many of the associated risk factors are still not fully understood. Because along with a number of lifestyle factors that can contribute to the development of diabetes, there are certain factors beyond one's control that can signal an increase risk. Each type of diabetes has its own set of risk factors, which we will go through one by one.

Nevertheless, these three factors apply to all types of diabetes:

- **Weight** - The increase in fatty tissue can make the cells more resistant to insulin. For women who plan on becoming pregnant, being overweight before pregnancy can increase the chances of gestational diabetes. Being overweight also makes diabetes more difficult to manage once diagnosed, can may just quicken the disease's progression.

- **Family history** - If you have a parent or sibling with

any type of diabetes, your risk for the disease increases. However, genetics is not destiny. In most cases, you can take measures to minimize your own likelihood of developing diabetes.

- **Inactivity** - Physical activity is integral to weight management. Exercising also uses up glucose as energy and makes the cells more sensitive to insulin.

Type 1 Diabetes Risk Factors

Although generally considered unpreventable, the following risk factors may contribute to a greater likelihood of one developing the Type 1 diabetes:

- **The presence of autoantibodies** - If Type 1 diabetes or any autoimmune disease runs in the family, you should consider getting tested for damaging immune cells, known as autoantibodies. Although it contributes to an increase risk, not everyone with autoantibodies develop diabetes.

- **Nutritional and dietary factors** - A diet low in vitamin D, early exposure to cow's milk formulas and cereals before 4 months of age are believed to increase the risk of Type 1 diabetes. None of these have been proven to be the direct cause though.

- **Geography and environmental factors** - It is likely that exposure to viral illnesses can play a role in Type 1 diabetes. According to the Mayo Clinic, a non-profit organization dedicated to clinical research, education and practice, Type 1 diabetes seems to be more prevalent in certain countries like Sweden and Finland. Exactly why that's the case remains unknown.

Prediabetes and Type 2 Diabetes Risk Factors

Generally regarded as both an inherited and lifestyle disease, many of the Type 2 diabetes risk factors can actually be reduced with knowledge and diligence. Even so, there are some factors we have less control over and would take more than a lifestyle adjustments to fix:

- **Age** - With each additional candle to the birthday cake, your metabolism slows down, making is easier to gain weight and lose muscle mass. Your immunity also weakens as the years take their toll on the body. Thus, plenty of risks for diseases increase, not just diabetes.

- **Ethnicity** - While it is still unclear why, Mayo Clinic reports that African Americans, Native Americans, Hispanics and Asian Americans are at higher risk of diabetes.

- **Hypertension** - Having blood pressure over 140/90 mm Hg is not only linked to an increase risk in stroke and heart disease, but also Type 2 diabetes. This is all the more reason to regularly have your blood pressure checked, since high blood pressure usually happens without symptoms.

- **Polycystic ovarian syndrome (PCOS)** - For women, having PCOS causes irregular menstrual periods, excess hair growth and weight gain. Not only does it increases the chances of developing Type 2 diabetes, it also puts a women at risk of gestational diabetes, should she gets pregnant.

- **Abnormal levels of cholesterol** - If your high-density lipoprotein (HDL, a.k.a. good cholesterol) is lower than optimal, it's a signal for Type 2 diabetes risk.

- **High levels of triglycerides** - Triglycerides are a type of fat (known as lipid) in the blood that the body uses for energy. If your levels are higher than 150 milligrams per deciliter (mg/dL), it should be cause for concern.

Gestational Diabetes Risk Factors

Although women are only at risk of developing gestational

diabetes during pregnancy, this type of diabetes shares many of the risk factors of Type 2. Moreover, gestational diabetes itself is a risk factor for developing Type 2 later in life. Here are a few more risk factors to watch out for:

- **Age of pregnancy** - Women who get pregnant over the age of 25 are at higher risk than those who opt to enter motherhood younger.

- **Personal history** - You are at greater risk, if you have prediabetes before getting pregnant. Same goes if one has any of the Type 2 diabetes risk factors pre-pregnancy.

- **Birthing history** - Women who had delivered to a large baby, weighing more than 9 pounds (4kg), or had unexplained still birth with previous pregnancies, may be more likely to have gestational diabetes.

Why Prevention Matters

It is not an overstatement to say that diabetes is a frightening and depressing disease. Once diagnosed, your whole lifestyle has to be adjusted to accommodate it. Foods you once enjoyed have become taboo. Your daily activities have to be planned around medication schedules and monitoring your blood sugar. Vacations cannot clash with doctor's appointment for a checkup and to medication supply top-up. You world is no longer the same.

Hence, it's not that unusual for a person to react with denial when first diagnosed with diabetes. It's depressing enough to have to come to terms that something is wrong with them, and they now have to take drastic actions to manage the disease, whether it is going on a weight loss and diet plan or taking shots for a hormone that the body is supposed to naturally produce. On top of that, they have to deal with the mountain of information about this condition they now have to live with - medications, regular visits to the doctor, monitoring blood sugar and what to or not to eat going forth - it can be can be overwhelming. They are also faced with the daunting possibilities of the complications that could develop and what would become of their life as a result. The stress of managing the condition alone can take its toll on an individual, making them feel isolated and burdensome towards friends and family. And in some cases, send them into a spiral of depression. The American Diabetes Association even reported that diabetics are among the group of individuals at risk of developing depression.

Depression is a serious mental health issue altogether. When deep depression sets in on people with diabetes, they would lose their zest for life altogether. They would gradually lose the enthusiasm and energy for the activities they once enjoyed. This could in turn lead to them neglecting to monitor their glucose, sleeping too much, skipping medication and - at worst - harbor suicidal thoughts. Anyone can suffer from depression, but the mental condition becomes deadlier with individuals dealing with a serious illness like diabetes.

For all those aforementioned reasons, the old adage that prevention is better than cure could not be more applicable.

With that said, diabetes prevention has to start with immediacy, ideally when you are in perfect health.

Can You Really Diabetes-Proof Your Life?

Let's be clear right from the get-go: there is no such thing as a fail-proof diabetes prevention plan. In many - if not most - instances, diabetes is hereditary. If you have an immediate family member with the disease, you are more predisposed to the condition than someone else on the same level of health and fitness who do not have the "diabetic genes". But as we've established, your genes doesn't spell your fate - it just means you have to be extra diligent with your well-being, if you want to maximize your chances of evading diabetes.

The problem is our modern lifestyle is getting increasingly more and more conducive to the development of diabetes. It's bad enough that processed food has become a mainstay in most households of many developed and developing economies. The working culture with lengthy hours being cooped up in the office, under fluorescent lights and staring at the computer screen has allowed little time for people to devote to their well-being. Then, there is the most overlooked component and also arguably the root of all health problems, big and small: emotional stress. Being under a lot of stress lowers your immunity, it contributes to weight gain and all sorts of ailments that turns the body's system into a breeding ground for all sorts of deadly diseases.

We tend to think of diabetics as people with a sweet tooth who lacked the self-control to curb their sugar cravings, but that could not be more further from the truth. In certain cases, diabetes still ends up developing despite one's best efforts, especially Type 1.
We know for a fact that out of the three main diabetes risk factors - weight, genetics and physical inactivity - we do have control over two of them. Thus, a sensible diabetes prevention plan will be revolved around the two key factors that are within our means to improve upon, which is by managing weight, through diet and regular exercise. So,

regardless of how high or low your risk may be, or even if you are diagnosed with prediabetes or one of the types of diabetes, all hope is not loss. With proper knowledge on what foods are good for you, and a willingness to get up and get moving, diabetes does not have to interfere with your quality of life.

When to see a Doctor

As much as we want to keep our focus on preventing diabetes altogether, we should not undermine possible early symptoms of the disease and the importance of physician care. It is possible to have diabetes with very mild to no symptoms. It is not too uncommon for people to develop diabetes and not know it for some time, until symptoms progress. Moreover, prediabetes that often leads to Type 2 has no symptoms at all. According to the International Diabetes Foundation, here are the symptoms that should be promptly checked:

Frequent urination and thirst

When your blood sugar is high, you will urinate more often, because when insulin is not doing its job, your kidneys cannot filter the glucose back into the blood. What happens is the kidneys will draw water from the blood to filter out and get rid of the excess glucose. Naturally, the more you urinate, the thirstier you will feel as you need to replace the lost fluid. We need eight to 10 glasses (up to 12 glasses, if the weather is hot and dry) of water each day to stay sufficiently hydrated. But if you find yourself with a full bladder often and need to drink more water due to insatiable thirst, something could be wrong.

Frequent hunger pangs

Because the body cells are not getting enough fuel due to lack of insulin, you may experience a sudden increase in appetite and feel hungrier faster after eating as a response to the body seeking out energy sources.

Unusual weight fluctuations

Constantly being hungry may lead to overeating and eventual weight gain. On the other hand, sudden unexplained weight loss and muscle wastage is also a sign not to be ignored. It is possible that because cells are getting the glucose they need for energy, muscle tissue and fat will be broken down as fuel supply. This kind of weight loss usually happens with Type 1, since the onset is more sudden, as opposed to Type 2 which develops gradually. Either way, sudden and unexplained weight fluctuations should not be dismissed.

Fatigue and irritability

When your body is not getting the fuel it needs, you will feel more tired, even with adequate sleep and calories. The lack of energy may make you irritable and listless.

More infections and slow healing wounds

Having more sugar in the blood lowers the body's resistance and ability to recover from all sort of physical injuries, like cuts and bruises. Open wounds and skin lesions would be more susceptible to infections. Your skin is also more prone to rashes and yeast infections. Due to anatomical structure, women in particular are at risk of vaginal and bladder infections that are difficult to recover from.

Gum Problems

Reddish, tender and swollen gums that pull away, making for loose the teeth - or any combination of these symptoms - may be a sign of diabetes. You may also experience gum disease and infections more often.

Signs of nerve damage

Too much blood sugar will gradually have an effect on your nervous system. Watch out for frequent numbness and tingling sensations in your limbs, especially the hands and feet. Another urgent sign from your body is blurred vision. Where the eyes are concerned, you want to quickly get checked for diabetes and get treatment before any long-term vision problems set in.

Diabetes can easily be detected by carrying out urine test to check for the presence of excess glucose. A diagnosis is normally confirmed with a follow-up blood test to measure glucose levels. If you or anyone you know may have the aforementioned symptoms that you suspect could have something to do with your metabolism, please do not take matter into your own hands and attempt to self-treat. See a doctor as soon as possible to get tested!

CHAPTER 3

WEIGHT MANAGEMENT MADE EASY

It should come as no surprise that obesity is responsible for many of the illnesses, and diabetes is just one of them. While staying slim and trim is no guarantee you will be disease-free, being overweight certainly sets you on a path towards becoming a ticking time bomb of illnesses, especially as you get older. Hence, maintaining an optimal body weight is not only crucial for preventing diabetes, but also in lowering your risk for a lot of other deadly diseases. Before we get into the details about eating right and exercising, let's go over the basics of what constitutes the ideal body weight. (Hint: it's not based on the images you see on TV and pages of glossy magazines!)

There are two indicators of whether one is of a healthy weight or not: body mass index (BMI) and waist circumference.

Calculating Your BMI

A healthy weight is one which is right for your height, based in your BMI. To calculate your BMI, find out your height in meters (m) and weight in kilograms (kg), then calculate using the following formula:

- Weight (kg) / Height (m)
- Divide the answer with you height (m) again, and that is your BMI

So, for example, if you weigh 65kg and measure at 1.70m in height:

- 65 / 1.70 = 38.2
- 38.2 / 1.70 = 22.5
- Your BMI is 22.5kg/m2

You are in a recommended weight range if your BMI is between 18.5 and 24.9. A BMI below 18.5 is considered underweight, which warrants a discussion with your doctor to check if your weight may be a symptom of a health condition.

A BMI of 25 to 29.9 qualifies as overweight, but is does not necessarily mean one is unhealthy. Body builders and athletes who trained to gain larger muscle mass may have a BMI that falls in the overweight category, which would be perfectly fine as long as they follow a good diet and maintains a higher muscle to fat ratio. If your BMI is 30 and above though, you are in the obese category and it is imperative that you start working on shedding the kilos!

It's worth bearing in mind that BMI is only one indicator of good health. You could have a BMI of 19 and still be setting yourself up for all sorts of disease if you do not eat well and exercise regularly. Nevertheless, if you find your clothes have become tighter and you are less energetic than you used to be, knowing your BMI gives you somewhere to start in taking charge of your health.

Your Waistline, Your Lifeline

The size of the waist circumference is perhaps more crucial than the BMI, and a more reliable predictor of one's bodily health. A person with a BMI within healthy range could have a weight circumference within the danger zone. It is a direct indicator of visceral fat, and carrying extra weight in the midsection lessens the body's ability to properly utilize insulin, thus leaving a buildup of glucose in the bloodstream.

To measure your waist circumference, wrap a measuring tape around your midsection first thing in the morning, right after you relief your bladder and before drinking water or having breakfast. For men, measurements should be taken at the belly button level. For women, take measurements at the smallest point where the waistline 'pinches' in. According to research by the Heart and Stroke Foundation, individuals of Caucasian, African, Middle-Eastern or Mediterranean descent are at increased risk of health issues if their waistline measurements exceed the following numbers:

- 109cm (40 inches) for men
- 88cm (35 inches) for women

Those of Far East, Southeast and South Asian descent, along with those of ethnic south and Central Americans, the ideal waist size for optimal health are:

- 91cm (36 inches) for men
- 81cm (32 inches) for women

The No Fuss Diet

There is no doubt about it that diet is an integral component to maintaining good health and keeping diseases at bay. You are what you eat! Alas, figuring out the right kind of diet is no easy task. If there is one subject experts in the health field have trouble agreeing on more than anything else, it's what constitutes the right diet. Take some time to look up articles in magazines, online and books written by credible sources, and you will most likely be stumped at what source or to whom you should listen to.

One doctor or dietitian may recommend an eating plan, only to have it criticized, disputed and contradicted by several others in the same field. Try asking for advice from your health-savvy and gym-going friends. One person could swear by complex carbs and high protein, while another may tell you to go fully vegan. Each would also most likely to be passionately trying to convince you of the merits of their dietary choices, and that you should make the switch if you want to be as healthy and disease-free as they are. It is no wonder - though strange as it may be - that people give up on being health conscious.

When it comes to eating for diabetes prevention and management, there are no shortage of diet plans endorsed by experts that would further add on to your confusion. Let's be clear; there is no such thing as a special anti-diabetic diet, despite the many types of eating plans you may have come across in the sea of information. All one has to do is follow a sensible and balanced diet, coupled with a practical exercise program, with the goal of attaining and maintaining optimal body weight. A healthy body weight goes a long way in keeping diabetes at bay - it is simple as that.

While the debate continues among proponents of specialty dietary plans on what constitutes a sensible diet, experts are generally in agreement on two points: you can't go wrong with a diet high in fiber, with plenty of vegetables, and cut down on processed food intake. With that in mind, let's keep it simple.

So, here's your anti-diabetes weight management plan in a nutshell:

- **Follow a sustainable eating plan** - A sensible healthy diet is one that you would not have trouble maintaining for the long-run. It is flexible and adaptable, based on simple and scientifically proven nutritional principles. No starvation, deprivation or restrictive eating. You should not be bored of your daily meals, because life is too short to not enjoy good food!

- **Avoid fad dieting** - Do not follow any eating plans that comes with a book of strict rules to follow, those that advocate eating only one type of food group, and promises rapid weight loss, with a celebrity endorsement thrown in for good measure. Many fad diets are based on meal plans that are almost impossible to keep up over a long period of time, and could do more harm than good. It's just not a balanced and healthy approached. Plenty of testimonies from fad dieters reported speedy weight loss, only to experience a rebound a few months later when they can no longer realistically follow the meal plan.

- **Maintain a diet consisting predominantly of plant sources** - You cannot go wrong with any food source that grows from the earth. The typical modern diet often lacks fruits and vegetables that are important sources of essential vitamins and minerals. Animal food sources do have their own nutrients as well, and becoming a vegetarian is a matter of personal choice.

Whatever the case, plant sources should be the dominant feature of your daily meals.

- **Portion control over calorie counting** - Always having to keep track of the amount of calories you are ingesting could work for people who are morbidly obese, and is in dire need to shed off pounds. Even so, it should be done under professional supervision. For regular people who just want to lose some weight and stay in shape, calorie counting fosters an obsessive attitude that might lead to more stress and possibly eating disorders. Instead of tracking calories, all you have to do is be mindful of your portion sizes. (More on portion control in Chapter 4)

- **Cut down on processed and junk food** - In a perfect world, you want to swear off processed and junk food for life, but we don't live in a perfect world. It may not be realistic to eliminate the processed stuff entirely from your diet, but you can at least try to cut them out by 90%. There's no harm in enjoying the occasional potato chips and soda, or have instant noodles for supper; just try to keep them to the minimum as possible. A simple tip to do this is by reaching for a healthier alternative. For example, if you want to have something to munch, you can opt for cashew nuts instead of potato chips. Go for fruit juice instead of carbonated soda.

- **Use the Glycemic Index (GI) principles as guidelines** - The glycemic index was developed to rank food depending on the rate which the body metabolizes it into glucose. Where diabetes is concerned, the GI is a wonderful guide for choosing the type of carbohydrates that are converted more slowly into energy by the body, thus avoiding sudden spikes in blood sugar. You will learn more about the GI and how it can be a wonderful guide to eating healthier in the next two chapters.

- **Get a minimum of 180-200 minutes of moderate-intensity exercise each week** - Exercise is an equally important component for weight management and minimizing the risks for diseases. More on exercising in Chapter 6.

There's nothing drastic and expensive that you need to do to start making the shift towards a healthier lifestyle that lowers your diabetes risk. If anything, all you really need is a willingness to start taking greater self-responsible towards your health and well-being. If diabetes runs in your family and you don't want that to be an inevitability for you, you are already in a good place to start minimizing your risk factors. To get yourself into the spirit of making a change, it is recommended that you start by weighing yourself, taking measurements of your waistline and then calculate your BMI. Do it the first thing in the morning after waking up, before breakfast for accuracy, then write it down. You don't have to do this at all, but if your goal is to lose weight - especially if it's the doctor's orders - it helps to measure your progress.

A note to those who plan on tweaking their diet for weight loss: do not get too caught up with the numbers on the scale.

Weighing and measuring yourself once a month should be enough.

CHAPTER 4

ALL YOU NEED TO KNOW ABOUT THE GLYCEMIC INDEX

There is no doubt that eating healthy is the key factor to disease prevention. Typically, that would mean knowing the nutritional value of the foods we eat, so that we are sure to get sufficient amounts of vitamins and minerals necessary for optimal bodily function. While this should certainly always be the case, there is one often overlooked component to a healthy diet: choosing the right kind of carbohydrate sources.

Carbohydrate food sources are very diverse and the body metabolizes them at different rates. Certain carbohydrates turn to sugar more than others. For instance, starches are especially slow to digest, and causes a higher rise in blood glucose. Hence, diabetics are often warned about watching their carbohydrate intake. It's impossible to eliminate carbohydrates from our diet altogether, nor is it encouraged. After all, we need the energy to function. So, what we can do is choose our carbohydrate sources wisely, and this is where the Glycemic Index (GI) comes in handy.

The GI is a concept developed by Dr. David J. Jenkins of the University of Toronto in 1981, with the purpose of measuring the effects of carbohydrates on blood sugar levels. This will give us an indication of how sugar is being used by the body. For diabetics and those with prediabetes, familiarizing oneself with the GI is important in order to understand how foods have an impact on your blood sugar. That doesn't mean its function is exclusive to combating and managing diabetes. Anyone can in fact use the GI as a tool to make informed lifestyle and dietary decisions. With diabetes becoming an epidemic around the world, there is no reason not to empower yourself by learning more about what goes into your body.

What the GI does is basically rate different carbohydrate food sources based on their effect on different levels of glucose, on a scale of 1 to 100. Foods that get broken down rapidly and thus cause less harm to the system are placed low on the GI. The carbs that take longer to digest are ranked higher. Basically, carb sources with a rating of 50 and below are considered low GI foods. Those that fall between 51 and 70 are considered medium, and anything above 70 are high in the GI.

Low vs. High GI

Here's a quick trivia: In between a bar of chocolate and baked potato, which food item ranked higher in the GI and is considered more harmful to your blood sugar? The typical knee-jerk answer would be a chocolate bar, which would be incorrect as it only reinforces the myth that sweets and snacks heightens your chances of getting diabetes.

Surprisingly, a chocolate bar is safer for your blood sugar as it has an average GI of only 51 (some higher or lower, depending on the type and brand). On the other hand, baked potato has a GI of 111, making it one of the slowest to metabolize foods! Simply put, a chocolate bar is a safer source of energy for diabetics and prediabetics than baked potatoes.

Take a moment and look at your own diet. Have you been getting your carbs mainly from high GI foods? Now that you know not all carbs are equal, not to mention the impact they can have on your health in the long run, perhaps it's time to be more aware of what you consume. If you have a high diabetes risk factor or have a loved one diagnosed with the disease, the GI comes very much in handy to help you sort out your carbohydrate sources. Learning to substitute high GI foods with those of a lower GI is the first step towards having a more nutritionally balanced diet.

Besides keeping your blood sugar levels healthy, going low GI will do your energy levels a world of good as well. You will feel more alert and energized throughout the day, no more sluggishness and feeling quick to hunger that resulted from consuming sugar rich foods that are high on the GI. That's because lower GI foods consist of mostly complex carbs, which create slow energy release that keeps you feeling full for longer between meals, thus preventing overeating. Simple carbs, on the other hand, are those food that get converted into sugar, giving you a short burst of energy that melts away quickly. For people with weight troubles who find a challenge to keep the pounds off, a low GI diet could be the missing piece.

Perhaps the best thing about a low GI diet is that it can be adopted by anyone. If you are perfectly healthy, it will make it easier for you to manage your weight, and further lowers your risk of developing diabetes. If you have prediabetes, it could be all you need to stop Type 2 diabetes dead on its tracks. For those who have been diagnosed with diabetes, a low GI diet has been known to provide relief from symptoms and slow down the disease's progression, elevating the quality of life for diabetic individuals. Pregnant women can follow a low GI diet to avoid gaining to much weight and prevent gestational diabetes. If you shop and cook for your whole family, imagine the enormous benefits to be had from getting young children started on good carbs.

The most important thing to remember is that the higher your blood sugar level, the more insulin your pancreas has to release to make sure your body cells get the energy it needs. When that process fails and a lot of glucose is left in the blood, hyperglycemia happens. But when there's a high amount of insulin released, it can cause a sudden drastic dip in glucose levels, resulting in the opposite condition known as hypoglycemia. When that happens, a diabetic person could go from feeling disproportionate thirst and the urge to urinate frequently to experiencing a low energy and sudden hunger. Hence why eating the right carbohydrates that are good for your metabolism is crucial.

To sum it up, here's a list of the numerous benefits of a low GI carb diet:

- Weight loss and better weight management
- Increase in insulin sensitivity

- Greater satiety effect after meals
- Less tendency to overeat
- Increased energy and muscular endurances
- Better control over diabetes
- Lower risk of heart diseases
- Reduction in bad cholesterol levels
- Better management of PCOS
- Prevents hyper- or hypoglycemia

The Carbohydrates Debate

The GI has been a staple with dietary recommendations for diabetes management and prevention. It is indeed a scientifically backed, tried-and-true, smarter way of consuming carbs that won't damage your metabolism. With that said, is the GI really a foolproof guide to carbohydrates?

Logically, a good diet based on the GI means to consume more food items with lower GI, while reducing intake of higher GI items in one's regular diet. Very easy, right? Turns out, that's not the entire story. To clarify this, let's have a better understanding of the two types of carbohydrates - complex and simple carbs.

Almost all carbohydrates get broken down by the body and turn into glucose (there are those which do not, but we will get to that in the next chapter). The difference between simple and complex carbs is their chemical structure, which determines how fast they are metabolized by the body. At some point, most of us were possibly taught to stick to complex carbs because it helps regulate appetite and help you stay slim, and eat less simple carbs because too much sugar is bad for you. Pretty straightforward, right? Well, not really either.

Simple carbohydrates are also known as simple sugars. According to the National Health Service (NHS), a public funded healthcare system in England, adults are advised to consume less than 70g of sugar for men and less than 50g for women. People with diabetes and those who are overweight should be limited to even lower amounts. Sugars are found in many natural food sources, including fruits and vegetables. In fact, some fruits ranked higher on the GI than starches, but that doesn't mean you need to cut down on them as they are good for you (more explanation on this in next chapter). On their own, sugars are empty calories, which mean calories that provide no nutrition aside from energy. And by now you should already know, sugars consumed raise your blood glucose levels quickly.

Normally, when you read and hear about eating more complex carbohydrates, what comes to mind is usually starches. That means white bread, pastries, rice, potato and pasta. In some cultures, starches are staple foods and the benefits can somewhat be substantiated. For instance, the rate of obesity is rather low in countries like China and Japan, where white rice is part of a daily meal. Obesity and heart diseases are also lower in Mediterranean countries where people consume more pastries and pastas, as oppose to North America where diabetes seems to be on a rise. The NHS even advices diabetics to base meals around starchy carbs. The problem with this is even low GI starches can have a pronounced effect on blood sugar levels, because as carbohydrates, starchy foods require the body to produce more insulin that fat or protein food sources does. Furthermore, researches have shown that greater insulin production increases the insulin resistance. This can be a problematic for those diagnosed diabetes who are trying to moderate their sugar consumption.

So, what's the solution? **Opt for whole grain and vegetable starches!** Not only do they provide you with the slow-release energy you need, they also provide you with fiber and plenty of essential nutrients. Plus, they ranked even lower on the GI compared to their refined carbohydrates counterpart. The next time you shop for starchy foods, go for the whole grain versions of those products - brown rice, whole wheat flour bread, wholegrain cereals and sweet potatoes.

But that's not all to it! Just based on the GI, we know what kind of foods can cause your blood sugar to spike quickly, but that's only one side of the story: **The Glycemic Load (GL).**

The Glycemic Load on your Blood Sugar

At its very basic, a GI value assigned to foods are based on the speed which those foods are broken down and cause a rise in blood sugar. What the GI doesn't tell you is how high your blood sugar could go when you actually eat those foods. For that - according to Harvard Medical School - we have to look at the **glycemic load (GL)**, which is determined by how much carbs is in a single serving.

So, for a more complete and accurate idea of how the foods you eat affect your blood sugar, you need to have two pieces of information:

- **The Glycemic Index (GI)** that determines **how fast** the food is converted into glucose, thus causing your blood sugar levels to go up. By now, you already know that low GI foods release glucose slowly, while high GI foods release glucose rapidly.

- **The Glycemic Load (GL)** that determines **the amount of glucose** the food will deliver. Low GL foods produce less glucose, while high GL foods produce more glucose.

Calculating the Glycemic Load

When you buy a food item for cooking that comes in a packet, look at the label for Carbohydrates per serving (in grams), and then find out what the GI for the item is. With that information, use the following formula to calculate its GL per serving:

Carbohydrates per serving (g) x GI / 100 = GL per serving

A food with a GL of 10 or less is considered low, a GL of 11 to 19 is medium, and above 20 would be considered high. How does this information apply to our daily dietary habits?

The next and final chapter will explain how you can incorporate more good carbohydrate sources into your daily meals, using the GI and GL as your guide. Read it thoroughly, go back to it as many times as necessary, and most importantly, put it into practice.

CHAPTER 5

MAKING SENSE OF CARBOHYDRATES

Before the GI and GL were founded, it was generally assumed that a healthy meal should consist of complex carbs and simple carbs are to be avoided as much as possible. Hence, a number of the somewhat outdated dietary advices for diabetes control involves eating meals based on starchy carbs. But we now know that many of the complex carbs with a low GI, when consumed regularly over long periods of time, can have an adverse effect on blood sugar. Moreover, a lot of fruits and vegetables - many of which are rich in vitamins and minerals that are good for you - rank very high on the GI and fall into the simple carbs category.

As an example, let's calculate the GL of watermelon. The GI for a watermelon is a high 80. The carbohydrates per serving - a serving would be about a sizable slice of the fruit - is 6g.

- 6g x 80 = 480
- 480/100 = 4.8

A slice of watermelon has a low GL of only 4.8. Compare that to a source of complex carbs like pasta, which carries a low GI of 50 and a high GL of 24. Obviously, you can't eat pasta on its own, so let's say you add cheese to the mix, the GI value of the meal becomes 65 while the GL is over 30!So, what does this mean?

It means if you eat a slice of watermelon, your blood glucose will rise quickly since it is simple sugar and you will get a boost of energy for a while before getting hungry and need to eat again. But at the same time, the quick-rising blood sugar caused by the watermelon is in a lesser amount and requires less insulin release to process, compared to that of a bowl of mac and cheese. In theory, this kind of goes against the advice that simple carbs are evil and need to be avoided. Clearly, not all simple sugars are bad for you, the same as not all complex carbs should be considered the go-to food for diabetes prevention. This also shows that GL is a more accurate and reliable representation of which carbohydrates are healthier for your blood sugar.

Portion Control Made Easy

You are now armed with the most fundamental facts about carbohydrates and how your body gets affected. You already know how to find out if a carbohydrate-rich food can be good or bad on your blood sugar, using the GI and GL. But in a full course meal, carbohydrates won't be the only food group on your plate - it shouldn't be, if you are aiming for balance in your diet. So, the question is how much of your meal should consist of carbohydrates? This brings us to the subject of portion control, a principle which has to go hand in hand with knowledge of the GI and GL.

Portion control is not just about how big of a size your meals are, but also the amount of each nutrient group there are in a serving. A balance meal should consist of equal amount of protein and carbohydrates, with plant sources making up half of the entire serving. The problem with our diet in general is that our meals typically consist of either too much carbohydrates or too much protein, while being severely lacking in vegetables and fruits. You just need to take a look at any restaurant menu to know this is true. If you order a serving of fish and chips, for instance, what you'll get is a fish fillet (protein), some fries (high GI carbs) and some vegetables on the side, no bigger than the size of your palm (sometimes all you get are green peas).

To remedy this situation, the nutrition experts at Harvard School of Public Health created a simple guideline known as the Healthy Eating Plate. Anyone who has ever done research into health dietary practices probably have at some point come across the Food Pyramid, the triangular diagram that shows how much from each basic food group we should eat every day. It was considered the most comprehensive dietary guide worldwide, since its introduction by the United Stated Department of Agriculture (USDA) in the early 1990s.The Plate came about later, as a visual aid to assist in the practical application of the principles of the food pyramid in meal planning.

In other words, the purpose of the Plate is to simplify the principles of the food pyramid and pictorially show the proportion of what one should eat for main meals on a daily basis. That way, we not only know how much to eat, but also the optimal amount of protein, carbohydrates, vegetables and fruits we should eat. Portion control has never been this easy!

Preparing a balanced meal based on the Healthy Eating Plate model is as easy as following the **quarter-quarter-half principle**:

Step 1: Using a 10 inches (25cm) plate, imagine there is a line that goes through the middle, dividing the serving space in half, and one half is divided in two. Now, there are three sections on a plate – two quarters and one half.

Step 2: Fill the first quarter of the plate is filled with a major carbohydrate source. The food groups that fall in this category include, rice, noodles, bread, cereals and wholegrain products. Remember to keep the GI and GL in mind! For diabetics, be sure to measure your blood sugar levels in accordance to your doctor's advice. This will help you keep track of how your body responds to carbohydrates. You can then make adjustments to this portion of your meals accordingly. Depending on your diabetes, you may need to lessen the carbs on your plate.

Step 3: Fill the second quarter with a protein source. This section is for the meats and beans. Fish, poultry, meat, eggs, nuts, legumes and tofu belong here.

Step 4: Fill the other half of the plate with vegetables and add one serving of fruit. This ensures a diet rich in fiber and all the essential vitamins and minerals. So, fill the largest portion of the plate with leafy greens and fiber-filled fruits such as apples, oranges, bananas and papaya.

Step 5: Finally, complete the meal by drinking a glass of water. Staying hydrated is just as important as eating a balanced diet. Although plain water is preferable, you can opt for unsweetened beverages or milk and milk products to accompany a meal.

And there you have it! The beauty of the Plate is that it can be adapted to suit almost any kind of cuisine, from any culture. You do not need to change your way of eating; just adjust the proportions of the basic food groups in what you normally eat in accordance with the quarter-quarter-half principle. Combine that with what you learned about GI and GL thus far, and you are already on the road to healthy eating.

For example, for a typical western meal, you can still have your fish and chips, but perhaps you want to substitute the French fries for baked potato and reduce the carbohydrates portion to be the same amount as the protein. Then, fill up half of the plate with a serving of salad (with a non-creamy, low-fat dressing, of course). If you accustomed to eating rice every day, you can certainly continue having rice dishes regularly, but adjust for adequate amounts of protein and plant sources.

In addition to balancing the food groups in your meals and watching how much you eat, here are a few more useful tips to avoid overeating:

- **Eat just enough to make you feel full, not stuffed.** You will know it when you get there; when you feel bloated and sluggish, as if your stomach can't handle taking any more food, it's time to stop. So, know your limits and stick to it.

- **Feel hunger for 15 to 30 minutes before eating the next full course meal**. That way, you know you are truly hungry and not turning to food for comfort from emotional distress.

- **Find a healthier outlet for emotional stress.** Some people have a tendency for emotional eating, where they turn to food - usually sugary and salty snacks - whenever they are stressed out. If that's the case with you, it's time to figure out a better coping mechanism. Here's a simple suggestion: exercise! (more on this in a while)

- **Learn to eat slower and avoid eating in a hurry**. Take time to really taste and chew your food properly before swallowing. You will feel fuller, and less likely to go for second helping. Properly chewed up food is also easier to digest. Best of all, when you take the time to savor each bite, you will enjoy your food even more. Try it! The experience is almost Zen-like.

Get Moving!

Given that diabetes is a metabolic disease, it make sense to be mindful of how the type of foods you consume can affect your body chemistry. We have looked extensively at the impact of diet on blood sugar. Hopefully, you have a newfound awareness of what you eat and have started taking the steps to change your eating habits for the better. There is one last key component to lowering your diabetes risk that you need to incorporate into your life immediately, if you haven't yet to do so, and that is physical activity.

While maintaining a good diet is important. Consuming calories - even good calories - while continue leading a sedentary lifestyle is the analogical equivalent to filling a car with the best fuel but keep it parked in the garage. Exercise is crucial for everyone. In terms of diabetes prevention, exercising plays an enormous part in managing your weight, improves mental health and improving insulin sensitivity. When you keep muscles active, the body can better eliminate blood sugar, thus it keeps your metabolism health just as it keeps you in shape.

Ideally, you want to clock in 200 minutes of moderate to high intensity formal exercise each week for weight maintenance and heart health. That is a little over three hours of time set aside specifically for working out over the course of seven days, whether it be at a gym, taking a yoga class or brisk walking around the block.

If you don't have the physical capacity to exercise for 200 minutes a week, do not force yourself. It could be age, fitness level or a medical condition that limits your mobility. Even if you are in good health, but haven't exercised for ages, resist signing up for a cross fit training package on impulse and going warrior mode, because you are risking injury by putting your body through vigorous exercise all of a sudden.

Coach, Not Coax, Yourself into Fitness

The best way to adopt a more active lifestyle is to do it gradually. Start small, so that you allow yourself to build the stamina and strength necessary, and then start to incorporate higher intensity exercises into your regimen.

If you are at loss of how to start exercising where to start, why not start with the most basic of exercises: walking? Many health professionals recommend walking 10,000 steps a day for weight maintenance and heart health. If you have been physically inactive thus far, chances are you won't make it to 10,000 steps at your first few tries. That's okay; don't beat yourself up over it. Just make it a point to take a stroll around the neighborhood either every morning before you go to work or in evening after you come back - whatever works for you. It doesn't have to be everyday either; just four days a week will do. That's already an hour of extra physical activity in your week. You can start with just 15 minutes. Do it every day to cultivate the habit, and then turn 15 minutes into 30 minutes, and eventually work up to an hour. When that feels too easy, add more days to the week. You may even want to invest in a pedometer to track your step count and aim for 10,000 steps per day. If you keep it up and stay dedicated, before you know it, you will notice an improvement in your stamina. Once you get there, you may then decide to invest in you fitness; get a gym membership, take up a sport or join a yoga studio.

No More Excuses!

The number one excuse people often come up with for not

exercising is time constraints. They have no time because they are too busy with work and family commitments. That should hardly be an excuse, because if one truly cares about their well-being they can always make room for exercising in their schedule. After all, nothing can buy you more than 24 hours a day; it's all a matter of how you choose to spend the hours available. You can sit before the TV with a bag of potato chips, or tend to your garden and work up a sweat. The point is, with a little bit of imagination, there are plenty of ways to get a little extra exercise into your daily routine. If a large chunk of your day is spent desk bound, any kind of extra physical activity to get you on your feet and have your heart pumping helps. And if you were to just take a moment to look at your daily routine, from the time you get out of bed to start the day until you retire at night, there are in fact plenty of things you can be doing as a workout.

Here are some ideas:

- Takes the stairs instead of the escalator whenever possible

- Cycle or walk instead of drive if you are going somewhere not too far from home and the weather is fine
- Do gardening and clean the house
- Walk the dog further than usual
- Dance!
- There are plenty of exercise routine videos on YouTube that you can do at home; give them a try

You have absolutely no legitimate excuse not to get up and moving.

What is Best for Me?

With all that you have learned about carbohydrates and what it can do to your blood sugar, the question becomes how do you even begin making the switch to a more sensible diet? There is actually no hard-and-fast rules when it comes to what you should and shouldn't eat. Sure, there are stuff that is bad for you, no matter what; processed food with refined sugars are definitely bad for you and should have little to no place in your regular diet.

Firstly, nutrition can be a complicated subject, as new researches and studies are continuously being done. Thus, it is no surprise that we constantly ended up with a plethora of confusing, often contradicting and sometimes even misleading information. What may be considered a "super food" for daily consumption could be known as the slow killer a few decades later.

Perhaps the best we can do for ourselves is to take whatever advice one can get from a reliable source, put them in practice and observe the results for ourselves to see if it actually works for you. That means we need to take responsibility for ourselves by being more aware of our well-being. After starting a new diet plan, pay attention to how you feel throughout the day. Do you have more energy than before? Are you more alert and able to better concentrate at work? Does it feel easier to make it through your workouts at the gym? Do you get sick less often? If weight loss is your goal, you want to be keeping an even closer eye on your progress from the time you implement a new diet plan.

Granted, this can be even trickier for diabetics, which is why it is imperative to closely monitor your blood sugar before and after a meal, and discuss with your doctor as you make adjustments to your diet. For those who have been diagnosed with diabetes or prediabetes, testing your blood sugar levels using a home test kit approximately two hours before and after meals is a good way to assess how much carbs your body can cope with.

The trial-and-error process of figuring what works for you and what doesn't can be frustrating in the beginning, but muster up some patience and don't give up on yourself. Plenty of studies and anecdotal evidence have shown that people who managed to successfully lose weight and keep it off did so with self-observation, continuous learning and figuring out their own body chemistry, and then make adjustments to their lifestyle accordingly. For example, endurance sport athletes and those who hold physical jobs would need more high GI foods, as opposed to those who works in an office.

It is highly encouraged that you keep a food log as you work on refining your diet. Write down everything you eat for breakfast, lunch, dinner and supper. Use your food log to plan grocery shopping and meals ahead of time. Getting into the habit of noting down what you eat gives you some sort of a road map, so that you can see if there is any noticeable patterns to the foods you tend to favor and makes you more conscious of how your body handle handles food. A food log also comes in handy to help you detect any abnormalities or sickness that may arise from something you eat. For diabetics, it is an indispensable tool to controlling the disease. So, in addition to keeping record of what you eat for the day, you want to note down your blood sugar test readings as well.

In the end, the right type of diet for you should be one which supplies you with the energy you need to go about your day, while benefiting your overall health.

Your Diabetes Control and Prevention Cheat Sheet

The full GI list is unfortunately beyond the scope of this book. There are numerous online and print sources that provide a comprehensive list of GI values for food groups, with some sources even list the carbohydrates per serving and GL. Look up a reliable source for a GI table and keep it around for reference. A good place to start is the website <u>mendosa.com</u> - one of the oldest and most comprehensive online resources for diabetes, with a listing of GI and GL for over 2000 foods.

Here is a guideline for how you can use knowledge of the GI and GL to your advantage, plus a number of useful tips and tricks. Consider this list a cheat sheet that you can quickly refer to for some helpful hints as you plan your meals.

Low GI and GL Foods:

There are the foods that should be a mainstay in your diet,

especially if you are diabetic or at a high risk.

- **Minimally processed whole grains** - Oats, brown rice, granola, muesli and whole-wheat pasta and whole-wheat bread
- **All non-starchy vegetables and leafy greens** - Broccoli, spinach, lettuce, onion, green peas and carrot
- **Most fruits with moderate to low amounts of natural sugar** - Citrus fruits, apples and berries
- **Plant protein sources** - Nuts, seeds, legumes and beans.
- **Organic raw yogurt and cheese** that are plain and unsweetened

High GI and GL Foods:

Most of these carbohydrates are good energy sources, when consumed in moderation, preferably the less sweetened option, and paired with low GI foods.

- **Starchy root vegetables** - Potatoes and squash, etc.
- **Refined grains and flour products** - Most bread,

breakfast cereals, cookies, pastries and cake
- **Natural sweeteners** - Maple syrup, molasses, raw honey, and table sugar
- **Dried fruits** - Plums, dates and raisins etc.

Bad High GI and GL Foods

With these foods, less is more, none is best.

- **Sweetened beverages** - Bottled juices, sparkling water and soda
- **Fast foods and deep fried foods** - The kind you usually buy from a drive-through
- **Empty calories** - What qualifies as empty calories are calories that have absolutely no nutritional value, but they do impact your blood sugar nonetheless. These are calories our bodies can do without as they only do you harm, without anything good. Alcohol and highly processed packaged foods that are loaded with artificial sweeteners fall into this category.

Best Foods to go with Carbohydrates

There is a GI and GL for pretty much every food item out there. However, there are some protein sources, oils and fats that contain no carbohydrates at all, and thus have a GI of 0. These types of foods should be an integral part in your daily meals.

Being smart with your choice of carbohydrates is one of the keys to a healthy metabolism, because every time you eat carbohydrate containing food, your blood sugar changes. Furthermore, it should also be noted that the GI and GL of foods changes depending on various factors, such as how it is cooked, what are the other ingredients added to them, how processed they, their fiber content and what other types of foods they are paired with in a meal serving.

These are the best foods to pair together with moderate serving of good carbs for regulating blood sugar and appetite, and also to give you more energy:

- **Fresh vegetables and whole pieces of fruits** - As explained in the segment on portion control, plant food sources should occupy the biggest space on your meal plate. Vegetables and fruits are best consumed fresh, because the heat from cooking can destroy or diminish some of their nutritional properties.
- **Quality protein** - Free-range eggs, grass-fed beef or mutton, wild fish and raw dairy products.
- **Healthy fats** - Extra virgin olive oil, virgin coconut oil, almonds, chia, flaxseed and avocado. Fishes are also good sources of healthy fats.
- **Healthy acids** - Apple cider vinegar, fermented yogurt, citrus juice and any vinegar-based salad dressing. These acidic foods have the benefit of lowering the GI of certain foods items.
- **High-fiber foods** - Leafy green vegetables, artichoke, flaxseed, beans, apples, pears, pumpkin seeds, almonds, oats and sweet potatoes.

Some additional meal preparation tips:

- **Low GI and GL whole grains are the best breakfast meal.** There is no better way to kick off your metabolism with a breakfast that will give you a greater satiety effect, so you have more energy, a more stable appetite and are less likely to eat a lot throughout the day. Don't skip breakfast; it is indeed the most important meal of the day!

- **Variety is the spice of life.** You probably have heard of so-called experts or celebrities (maybe some of your friends and family members) swearing by diet plans that involve eating only one category or type of food. These types of diets make you sick and tired of your meals, eventually caving in and give up on trying to maintain a healthy lifestyle. Not only that, you are simply not eating a balanced diet, because you are depriving yourself of certain nutrients.

- **Eat from nature.** In the world we live in today, it's an uphill battle to avoid processed foods. So, the goal is to minimize them in your daily intake. The best way to go about this is to select good ingredients and cook your meals yourself. When you eat out a lot, you don't really know what goes into the meal that's being served to you.

- **Baked is always better than fried.** Few of us can resist a scrumptious and savory bite, but fried foods absorb the fat from the oils. Consume a lot of fried foods and you are on your way to gaining weight. If you want to enjoy the occasional French fries, fry them yourself with olive oil, or opt for spiced baked potato wedges.

- **Pick healthy stuff to snack on.** Too much chips, candies, sweets and chocolates are just as bad for your blood sugar as they are for your teeth. If you want to have something to munch between meals, instead of those stuff filled with processed sugars, go for healthier snacks like nuts, whole grain crackers, dark chocolate and fresh fruits. Instead of a can of soda, squeeze yourself a glass of fresh fruit juice.

- **Low fat is not really your friends.** It seems like a no-brainer, right? If you want to keep the pounds off, just opt for low-fat alternatives to high-caloric and carbohydrates rich foods. Well, not really. The problem with low fat products - most notably milk and dairy - is that many of them have added sugar, salt preservatives and other unnatural additives to replace fat. Some of these foods also have their natural nutrient components tempered with or removed. Plus, plenty of research has shown that there is nothing unhealthy about full fat dairy. If anything, it is healthier. The rule of thumb is if it is made in a food manufacturer's lab and not found in nature, it has not place in your diet.

- **Artificial sweeteners aren't good for you either.** The American Heart Association (AHA), American

Diabetes Association (ADA) and the Food and Drug Administration (FDA) had all given the nod for using artificial sweeteners as a measure to combat obesity, metabolic diseases and diabetes. However, the truth is less clear cut. Experts are concerned over the long term effects of routinely using artificial sweeteners has on the way we taste food. These type of sweeteners are far more potent than natural ones. A tiny amount of it is enough to produce the intense sweet taste comparable to natural sugars, but without the equal amount of calories. This can lead to overstimulating the sugar receptors in the taste buds, causing one to become less tolerant to complex flavors. Eventually, fruits, vegetables and unsweetened foods becomes less palatable. In other words, you may end up shunning filling and highly nutritious foods in favor of artificially sweetened and less nutritional foods. There is a psychological side effect to adopting artificial sweeteners too; people tend to replace lost calories with other food sources, thinking that "If I'm drinking diet soda, it should be okay for me to have a second helping of cake".

- **Make it a habit to read food labels.** That small table on food packages that lists the percentage of all nutrients contained in the whole pack and per serving has all the valuable information you need. Never buy anything for consumption without checking the nutritional value as printed on the label.

- **Keep it simple.** The bottom line when it comes to deciding what kind of foods are good for you it to go by common sense and a bit of intuition. And whenever in doubt, always go with least processed and most natural options.

CONCLUSION

The very thought of making lifestyle changes may come across as a daunting task. You might be thinking, hold on...isn't this diabetes prevention plan supposed to be no hassle, no fuss? Why do I have to concern myself with things like high GI and low GI foods? - you may wonder, because the last thing you want is to get mathematical with your meals. Well, let's be upfront; when you consider any kind of lifestyle changes, there is obviously a learning curve and a period of adjustment. Whether it is easy or difficult, that depends entirely on the individual.

When you have chosen to make a change in the way you eat, you will need to reduce and even give up on certain foods that you are used to. This is necessary if you want to reap the rewards in the long-run. The initial changes may take some time to get used to.

Once you begin to, not only notice, but also feel a surge in your energy levels, how your mind and body functions better, and your zest for life rekindled, you will be thanking yourself for taking the initiative to improve your life.

It should be reiterated at this point that your diabetes prevention plan is not meant to get you preoccupied with keeping tabs on your meals, and definitely not to take away your enjoyment of food. You are just eliminating and replace carbohydrates that are bad for your metabolism. All that is asked of you here is to take a little bit of your time to learn and familiarize yourself with the GI and GL, so that you make smarter choices with your carbohydrate food sources when planning your meals.

As you put knowledge into practice, it eventually becomes a natural way of life. Before you know it, you will not shop for groceries, cook and eat out the same way you used to. You will become more conscious of what goes into your body, because as the old saying goes, you are what you eat. This in turn will see your risk for diabetes and other deadly diseases that come with age and weight gain significantly lowered.

Do not wait until orders to make healthier lifestyle choices are given by a doctor. With diabetes reaching epidemic levels, it is never too late to begin a prevention plan now.